Yoga Essentials

All you need to know about yoga, the importance,benefits and yoga poses

Jeff Anderson

TABLE OF CONTENT

Chapter 1: Introduction to Yoga

Chapter 2: The Importance of Yoga

Chapter 3: Benefits of Yoga

Chapter 4: Getting Started with Yoga

Chapter 5: Yoga Poses for Beginners

Chapter 6: Intermediate and Advanced Yoga Poses

Chapter 7: Creating Your Yoga Routine

Chapter 8: Beyond the Mat – Integrating Yoga into Daily Life

Conclusion: A Lifelong Journey of Yoga

Chapter 1

Introduction to Yoga

The Rich Tapestry of Yoga

In the quiet corridors of ancient wisdom, yoga emerged as a profound practice that transcends the boundaries of time and culture. Rooted in the spiritual traditions of ancient India, yoga is a holistic approach to harmonizing the mind, body, and spirit. As we embark on this journey into the heart of yoga, let us unravel the rich tapestry that makes this practice a timeless beacon of well-being.

A Glimpse into the Past

Yoga's origins can be traced back thousands of years, finding its first expressions in the Vedas and Upanishads. These sacred texts laid the foundation for a system that seeks to unite individual consciousness with universal consciousness. Over the centuries, different schools of thought have woven their interpretations into the fabric of yoga, each contributing to its diverse and inclusive nature.

Philosophy and Mind-Body Connection

At its core, yoga is more than a physical exercise; it is a philosophy that emphasizes the interconnectedness of all aspects of life. The word "yoga" itself is derived from the Sanskrit word "yuj," meaning to yoke or unite. This union refers to the integration of mind, body, and spirit, fostering a profound sense of harmony and balance.

Cultural Roots and Global Impact

While yoga originated in ancient India, its teachings have traversed continents, cultures, and centuries. Today, yoga is a global phenomenon, embraced by people seeking not only physical fitness but also mental clarity and spiritual insight. From bustling urban studios to serene mountain retreats, the practice of yoga continues to evolve, adapting to the needs of diverse communities.

Mindfulness and Present Moment Awareness

One of the foundational principles of yoga is mindfulness—the art of being present in the moment. In a world often marked by chaos and distraction, yoga provides a sanctuary for individuals to turn inward, cultivating a heightened awareness of their thoughts, emotions, and physical sensations.

As we delve deeper into the chapters that follow, let this introduction serve as a gateway to the transformative power of yoga. We will explore its importance, delve into the myriad benefits it offers, and guide you through the essential yoga poses that form the building blocks of this ancient practice. Join us on this journey as we unlock the secrets of yoga and discover its profound impact on our holistic well-being.

Chapter 2

The Importance of Yoga

Nurturing the Body, Mind, and Soul

Having traversed the historical corridors of yoga's origins, we now turn our focus to the present—the significance of yoga in our modern lives. Yoga, in its multifaceted glory, offers a myriad of benefits that extend far beyond the confines of a yoga mat. In this chapter, we explore the importance of integrating yoga into our daily routines, unraveling the transformative power it holds for our overall well-being.

Physical Harmony

In a world marked by sedentary lifestyles and constant digital engagement, the importance of physical activity cannot be overstated. Yoga, with its gentle yet powerful postures, becomes a sanctuary for those seeking to nurture their bodies. It enhances flexibility, builds strength, and improves balance—foundational elements for a healthy and resilient physique.

Mental Resilience

The demands of modern life often create a barrage of stress and anxiety. Yoga, with its emphasis on mindful breathing and meditation, becomes a refuge for cultivating mental resilience. By engaging in the present moment, practitioners learn to navigate life's challenges with a calm and centered mind, fostering emotional well-being.

Spiritual Connection

Beyond the physical and mental realms, yoga invites us to explore our spiritual dimensions. It provides a sacred space for self-discovery and reflection, offering a path to connect with a deeper sense of purpose and meaning. The journey within becomes as essential as the physical postures, as we tap into the wellspring of inner wisdom.

Balancing the Energies

Central to yogic philosophy is the concept of balancing the energies within the body. Through the practice of specific postures and breathwork, yoga aims to harmonize the vital life forces, or "pranas," promoting overall vitality and a sense of equilibrium. This balance extends beyond the mat, influencing our interactions and relationships.

A Holistic Approach to Well-Being

What sets yoga apart is its holistic approach to well-being. It acknowledges the interconnectedness of the body, mind, and soul, recognizing that true health is a harmonious integration of these elements. As we delve into the benefits of yoga in the next chapter, we will witness how this holistic perspective unfolds in myriad ways, touching every facet of our lives.

In the chapters that follow, we embark on a journey into the heart of yoga's benefits, exploring how this ancient practice has the potential to transform not just our bodies, but our entire way of being. Join us as we uncover the layers of significance that make yoga an indispensable companion on the path to holistic wellness.

Chapter 3

Benefits of Yoga

A Tapestry of Wellness Unveiled

As we stand at the threshold of understanding the importance of yoga, it is time to unfurl the vibrant tapestry of benefits that this ancient practice weaves into the fabric of our lives. Yoga is more than a series of physical postures; it is a holistic approach to well-being that extends its benevolent touch to every corner of our existence.

Physical Flourishing

The physical benefits of yoga are both tangible and transformative. Regular practice enhances flexibility, allowing the body to move with grace and ease. Strength is cultivated through asanas, fostering stability and resilience. Balance, both literal and metaphorical, becomes a natural outcome, influencing how we navigate the challenges of daily life.

Mental Clarity and Emotional Harmony

The practice of yoga is a sanctuary for the mind, offering a respite from the cacophony of modern existence. Mindful breathing and meditation techniques infuse a sense of calm and focus, empowering practitioners to navigate the complexities of their thoughts and emotions. The result is mental clarity, emotional resilience, and a greater capacity for joy.

Stress Reduction and Relaxation

In the hustle and bustle of contemporary life, stress has become an unwelcome companion. Yoga provides an antidote, offering a space for intentional relaxation and stress reduction. Savasana, the final resting pose, becomes a sacred moment to surrender, letting go of tension and embracing a state of profound relaxation.

Enhanced Respiratory Function

Breath, the life force that sustains us, takes center stage in the practice of yoga. Pranayama, the art of breath control, not only deepens the connection between body and mind but also enhances respiratory function. Conscious breathing improves lung capacity, increases oxygen intake, and promotes overall respiratory health.

Holistic Health and Well-Being

Yoga's unique proposition lies in its ability to address the holistic nature of health. By integrating physical postures, breathwork, and mindfulness, yoga becomes a comprehensive tool for enhancing overall well-being. The benefits extend beyond the physical and mental realms, seeping into the very essence of our being.

A Fountain of Youth

As we explore the diverse benefits of yoga, it becomes evident that this practice has the power to turn back the hands of time. Through mindful movement, breath awareness, and the cultivation of a positive mindset, yoga becomes a fountain of youth—nourishing the body, invigorating the mind, and fostering a timeless sense of vitality.

In the forthcoming chapters, we embark on a journey into the heart of yoga's practice. We delve into the essential poses that form the foundation of this transformative art. Each pose, a gateway to physical and mental flourishing, carries within it a wealth of benefits waiting to be discovered. Join us as we navigate the landscape of 100+ yoga poses, unlocking the potential for holistic well-being that lies within each graceful movement and intentional breath.

Chapter 4

Getting Started with Yoga

Embarking on Your Yoga Journey

Now that we've explored the profound benefits of yoga, it's time to embark on the practical aspects of beginning your yoga journey. Whether you're a curious beginner or someone returning to the practice, this chapter will guide you on how to step onto the mat with intention and mindfulness.

Setting Your Intention

Begin your yoga journey with a clear intention. What brings you to the mat? Is it a desire for physical fitness, stress relief, or a journey of self-discovery? Setting a clear intention can anchor your practice, providing focus and purpose.

Choosing the Right Yoga Style

Yoga comes in various styles, each with its unique focus and pace. Explore different styles such as Hatha, Vinyasa, Ashtanga, or Yin to find the one that resonates with you. Some styles emphasize physical postures, while others focus on breathwork or meditation.

Experiment until you discover the style that aligns with your goals.

Finding a Suitable Class or Instructor

Whether in-person or online, finding the right yoga class or instructor is crucial. Look for classes tailored to beginners, and instructors who emphasize proper alignment and encourage a positive and inclusive environment. Attend a variety of classes to discover different teaching styles.

Investing in Essential Yoga Gear

Yoga doesn't require a vast array of equipment, but a few essentials can enhance your practice. Invest in a quality yoga mat that provides stability and comfort. Comfortable clothing that allows for free movement and a water bottle are also valuable additions to your yoga gear.

Understanding Basic Etiquette

Yoga classes often follow a set of unwritten etiquettes that contribute to a harmonious practice environment. Arrive on time, set up your mat mindfully, and avoid wearing strong scents. Most importantly, be respectful of the space and energy of those around you.

Building Consistency

Consistency is key in yoga. Start with a realistic commitment, whether it's a few minutes each day or a couple of classes per week. As you build consistency, you'll begin to notice the cumulative benefits of your practice.

Listening to Your Body

Yoga is a personal journey, and it's crucial to listen to your body. Honor its limitations, embrace its strengths, and avoid pushing yourself into discomfort or pain. Yoga is not a competition; it's a practice of self-awareness and self-care.

Seeking Guidance for Modifications

If you have specific health concerns or physical limitations, don't hesitate to seek guidance from a qualified instructor. They can provide modifications and adjustments to ensure that your practice is safe and beneficial for your individual needs.

Mindful Progression

Yoga is a journey of continuous learning and growth. Celebrate your progress, no matter how small, and avoid comparing yourself to others. Embrace the process, and let each moment on the mat contribute to your overall well-being.

As you take your first steps into the world of yoga, remember that your practice is uniquely yours. With an open heart and a receptive mind, you'll find that yoga is not just a physical exercise; it's a transformative journey that unfolds with each breath and each movement. In the chapters that follow, we dive into the heart of the practice—exploring the fundamental yoga poses that lay the groundwork for physical and mental flourishing. Join us as we unlock the secrets of these poses and guide you through the art of mindful movement.

Chapter 5

Yoga Poses for Beginners

Foundation Stones of Your Yoga Practice

With a solid understanding of the foundational aspects of yoga, we now embark on the exploration of essential yoga poses. These poses serve as the building blocks of your practice, cultivating strength, flexibility, and balance. Whether you're new to yoga or looking to refine your foundation, this chapter will guide you through key poses with step-by-step instructions and insights.

Mountain Pose (Tadasana)

1. Starting Position: Stand tall with your feet hip-width apart, arms by your sides.

2. Alignment: Engage your thighs, lift your chest, and reach your arms overhead with palms facing each other.

3. Benefits: Improves posture, strengthens legs and core, and promotes grounding and stability.

Downward-Facing Dog (Adho Mukha Svanasana)

1.   Starting Position: Begin on your hands and knees with wrists under shoulders and knees under hips.

2.   Alignment: Lift your hips toward the ceiling, straighten your legs, and press your heels toward the floor.

3.   Benefits: Stretches the spine, hamstrings, and shoulders; strengthens arms and legs; energizes the entire body.

Warrior I (Virabhadrasana I)

1.	Starting Position: From Mountain Pose, step one foot back, keeping the front knee bent and the back leg straight.

2.	Alignment: Square your hips to the front, reach your arms overhead, and gaze forward.

3.	Benefits: Strengthens legs and core, opens the chest and shoulders, builds focus and determination.

Tree Pose (Vrikshasana)

1.	Starting Position: Stand on one leg, bringing the sole of the other foot to the inner thigh or calf.

2.	Alignment: Find a focal point, lift your arms overhead, and press your palms together.

3. Benefits: Enhances balance and concentration, strengthens legs, opens hips, and promotes a sense of rootedness.

Child's Pose (Balasana)

1. Starting Position: Kneel on the mat, sit back on your heels, and extend your arms forward.

2. Alignment: Rest your forehead on the mat, keep your arms extended, and relax in this resting position.

3. Benefits: Relieves stress and fatigue, stretches the back, hips, and thighs, promotes relaxation.

Cobra Pose (Bhujangasana)

1.   Starting Position: Lie on your stomach, place your hands under your shoulders, and lift your chest.

2.   Alignment: Keep your elbows slightly bent, engage your back muscles, and lift your gaze.

3.   Benefits: Strengthens the spine, opens the chest and shoulders, improves posture, and alleviates back pain.

Seated Forward Bend (Paschimottanasana)

1.   Starting Position: Sit on the mat with your legs extended in front of you.

2.   Alignment: Hinge at your hips, reach forward toward your toes, and lengthen your spine.

3.   Benefits: Stretches the spine, hamstrings, and lower back, calms the mind, and improves digestion.

Corpse Pose (Savasana)

1.   Starting Position: Lie on your back, arms by your sides, palms facing up, and legs extended.

2.   Alignment: Close your eyes, relax your entire body, and focus on your breath.

3.   Benefits: Promotes relaxation, reduces stress, and allows for integration of your practice.

As you familiarize yourself with these foundational poses, approach each with mindfulness and patience. The beauty of yoga lies not only in the physical postures but in the journey of self-discovery that unfolds with consistent practice. In the chapters ahead, we delve into more poses, gradually expanding your repertoire and deepening your connection to the transformative power of yoga. Join us on this exploration of movement, breath, and self-awareness.

Chapter 6

Intermediate and Advanced Yoga Poses

Elevating Your Practice

As your journey through yoga progresses, so does your capacity for exploration and growth. In this chapter, we delve into intermediate and advanced yoga poses, offering you the opportunity to elevate your practice to new heights. Remember, the key is not perfection but the continual expansion of your physical and mental boundaries.

Plank Pose (Phalakasana)

1.   Starting Position: Begin in a push-up position with your wrists under your shoulders.

2.   Alignment: Keep your body in a straight line from head to heels, engage your core, and hold.

3.   Benefits: Strengthens the core, shoulders, and arms, improves posture, and enhances overall stability.

Crow Pose (Bakasana)

1.   Starting Position: Squat down, place your hands on the mat shoulder-width apart, and bend your elbows.

2. Alignment: Lift your feet off the ground, bringing your knees to the backs of your arms, and balance.

3. Benefits: Strengthens the arms and wrists, tones the abdominal muscles, and improves concentration.

Wheel Pose (Urdhva Dhanurasana)

1. Starting Position: Lie on your back, bend your knees, and place your hands by your ears.

2. Alignment: Press into your hands and feet, lifting your hips and chest toward the ceiling.

3. Benefits: Opens the chest and shoulders, strengthens the arms and legs, and boosts energy.

Headstand (Sirsasana)

1. Starting Position: Kneel on the mat, interlace your fingers, and place the crown of your head on the floor.

2. Alignment: Lift your hips, straighten your legs, and find balance on the crown of your head.

3. Benefits: Enhances focus and concentration, strengthens the shoulders and core, and invigorates the entire body.

Pigeon Pose (Eka Pada Rajakapotasana)

1. Starting Position: From a downward-facing dog, bring one knee

toward your wrist and extend the other leg back.

2. Alignment: Square your hips, lower your chest toward the mat, and find a comfortable stretch.

3. Benefits: Opens the hips, stretches the thighs and groin, and releases tension in the lower back.

Extended Triangle Pose (Utthita Trikonasana)

1. Starting Position: Stand with your legs wide apart, arms parallel to the floor.

2.   Alignment: Hinge at your hips, reach one hand toward the floor, and extend the other arm upward.

3.   Benefits: Strengthens the legs and core, stretches the hamstrings and hips, and improves overall balance.

Firefly Pose (Tittibhasana)

1.   Starting Position: Squat down, place your hands on the floor between your feet, and straighten your legs.

2.   Alignment: Shift your weight forward, lift your hips, and extend your legs parallel to the ground.

3.   Benefits: Strengthens the arms, wrists, and core, improves balance, and challenges the entire body.

King Pigeon Pose (Rajakapotasana)

1.   Starting Position: Begin in a downward-facing dog, bring one knee toward your wrist, and extend the opposite leg back.

2.   Alignment: Reach back with your hand to grasp the foot, lifting the chest and opening the heart.

3.   Benefits: Stretches the thighs and hip flexors, opens the chest, and promotes emotional release.

As you explore these intermediate and advanced poses, approach them with humility and a sense of curiosity.

Consistent practice and patience will allow you to gradually integrate these poses into your repertoire. Remember, yoga is a continuous journey of self-discovery and growth. In the upcoming chapters, we'll further explore the nuances of your yoga practice, guiding you through sequences, mindfulness, and the integration of yoga into your daily life. Join us as we continue to unveil the transformative power of this ancient art.

Chapter 7

Creating Your Yoga Routine

Crafting Harmony in Movement

With a repertoire of foundational and advanced poses, it's time to weave them into a cohesive yoga routine. Creating a personalized routine allows you to tailor your practice to your individual needs, goals, and the time you have available. Let's embark on the journey of crafting a harmonious and balanced yoga routine.

Setting Your Intention

Begin your routine by setting a clear intention for your practice. Reflect on what you hope to achieve—whether it's physical strength, mental clarity, or emotional balance. Let your intention guide the energy and focus of your practice.

Warm-Up Sequence

Start with a gentle warm-up to prepare your body for more dynamic movement. Incorporate flowing movements, such as sun salutations, to awaken your muscles, increase circulation, and sync your breath with movement.

Foundation Poses

Integrate foundational poses into your routine to establish stability and alignment. Include a mix of standing poses, seated poses, and gentle stretches to target different muscle groups and ensure a well-rounded practice.

Progressive Sequences

Build on the foundation by incorporating progressive sequences. Link poses together in a flowing manner, allowing your movements to be guided by your breath. This not only enhances the physical challenge but also cultivates mindfulness and a meditative flow.

Balance and Inversion Poses

Include balance poses and inversions to challenge your stability and build strength. Poses like Tree Pose, Warrior III, and Headstand can be integrated strategically to enhance both physical and mental focus.

Flexibility and Stretching

Dedicate a portion of your routine to deep stretching and flexibility. Poses like Pigeon Pose, Seated Forward Bend, and

Cow Face Pose help release tension, improve flexibility, and enhance the range of motion in your joints.

Mindful Cool Down

As you approach the end of your routine, transition into a mindful cool down. Incorporate seated or reclined poses, allowing your body to relax and your mind to find stillness. Close your practice with a few moments of meditation or conscious breathing.

Restorative Poses

Include restorative poses, such as Child's Pose or Legs Up the Wall, for a soothing conclusion to your routine. These poses promote relaxation, release accumulated tension, and encourage a sense of calm.

Closing Meditation

Conclude your routine with a brief meditation or mindfulness practice. This allows you to absorb the benefits of your practice, center your mind, and carry the sense of calm and clarity into your daily life.

Reflect and Adjust

After each practice, take a moment to reflect on how you feel physically, mentally, and emotionally. Pay attention to what worked well and where you faced challenges. Use this feedback to adjust and refine your routine over time.

Remember, your yoga routine is a dynamic and evolving aspect of your practice. Feel free to modify and adapt it based on your evolving needs and goals. As we move forward, we'll explore the integration of yoga principles into your daily life, fostering a holistic approach to well-being beyond the confines of the mat. Join us in discovering how yoga becomes a way of living, breathing, and being.

Chapter 8

Beyond the Mat – Integrating Yoga into Daily Life

Living Yoga Off the Mat

As you delve deeper into your yoga practice, it's essential to recognize that the benefits of yoga extend far beyond the confines of the mat. This final chapter explores how you can integrate yoga principles into your daily life, fostering a holistic approach to well-being in mind, body, and spirit.

Mindful Breathing Throughout the Day

Bring the awareness of your breath into your daily activities. Whether you're at work, commuting, or engaged in routine tasks, practice conscious breathing. Inhale deeply, exhale completely, and cultivate a sense of presence in each moment.

Mindful Eating

Approach meals with mindfulness. Pay attention to the colors, textures, and flavors of your food. Chew slowly and savor each bite. Eating mindfully not only enhances digestion but also cultivates a deeper connection with the nourishment your body receives.

Yoga in Movement

Incorporate simple yoga stretches into your daily routine. Whether you're waiting in line, sitting at your desk, or taking a break, perform gentle stretches to release tension and maintain flexibility. These mini yoga breaks contribute to overall well-being throughout the day.

Mindful Communication

Apply the principles of yoga to your interactions with others. Practice active listening, speak with kindness, and cultivate compassion. Yoga teaches us the importance of connection, and mindful communication fosters harmonious relationships in all aspects of life.

Gratitude Practice

Take a moment each day to express gratitude. Reflect on the positive aspects of your life, acknowledging the blessings, no matter how small. A gratitude practice fosters a positive mindset, leading to a more joyful and fulfilling life.

Digital Detox and Mindfulness

In a world dominated by screens and constant connectivity, practice digital detoxing. Set aside dedicated periods each day to disconnect from electronic devices. Use this time for self-reflection, meditation, or simply to enjoy the beauty of the present moment.

Yoga Philosophy in Decision-Making

Apply the ethical principles of yoga, such as the Yamas and Niyamas, to your decision-making process. Consider concepts like non-violence, truthfulness, and contentment as guiding principles in your actions. This approach promotes ethical and conscious living.

Self-Care Rituals

Incorporate self-care rituals into your routine. Whether it's a soothing bath, a walk in nature, or moments of quiet reflection, prioritize activities that nourish your mind, body, and soul. Self-care is an essential aspect of the yoga lifestyle.

Connection to Community

Yoga emphasizes the interconnectedness of all beings. Foster a sense of community and connection with others. Engage in acts of kindness, volunteer, or participate in group activities that align with your values. Creating a supportive community enhances the sense of belonging and purpose.

Continued Learning and Growth

Embrace a mindset of continuous learning and personal growth. Explore new aspects of yoga, delve into related subjects, and seek opportunities for self-improvement. The journey of yoga is a lifelong exploration that evolves with your experiences and insights.

As you integrate these yoga principles into your daily life, you'll find that the practice becomes a way of living—a holistic and transformative approach to well-being. Beyond the physical postures, yoga becomes a guiding philosophy, offering a path to a more conscious, balanced, and fulfilling existence. May your journey off the mat be a source of inspiration, growth, and profound connection.

Conclusion

A Lifelong Journey of Yoga

Congratulations on reaching the culmination of this journey into the heart of yoga! As you reflect on the principles, poses, and practices shared in this book, remember that yoga is not a destination but a lifelong journey of self-discovery, growth, and well-being.

Embracing the Essence of Yoga

Yoga is a versatile and adaptable practice that extends its transformative touch to every aspect of your life. It's more than a series of physical postures; it's a philosophy that invites you to explore the depths of your mind, the resilience of your body, and the expansiveness of your spirit.

Continual Exploration and Evolution

As you continue your yoga journey, remain open to exploration and evolution. Your practice will naturally evolve with your changing needs, experiences, and understanding. Embrace new challenges, welcome different styles of yoga, and let your practice reflect the dynamic nature of your being.

Mindful Living in Every Breath

In the hustle and bustle of daily life, let the mindfulness cultivated on the mat infuse each breath. Use the lessons learned in yoga to navigate challenges, cultivate gratitude, and savor the richness of each moment. The practice of yoga is not confined to a specific time or space; it's a way of living mindfully in the present.

The Harmony of Mind, Body, and Spirit

Yoga is a harmonious union of mind, body, and spirit. Allow this integration to guide your choices, actions, and relationships. As you find balance on the mat, let it translate into a balanced and harmonious life off the mat—a life aligned with your truest self.

Sharing the Gift of Yoga

As you reap the rewards of your yoga journey, consider sharing this transformative gift with others. Whether by teaching, practicing kindness, or simply being a source of inspiration, you contribute to the collective well-being of the world. The ripple effect of your positive energy can create a more compassionate and connected community.

Gratitude for the Journey

Express gratitude for the journey you've undertaken. Whether you're a novice or an experienced yogi, each step on this path contributes to your growth and well-being. Cherish the moments of stillness, the challenges overcome, and the joy discovered through the practice of yoga.

A Lifelong Companion

Yoga is not a practice reserved for a specific phase of life—it is a lifelong companion. It evolves with you, offering solace in times of challenge and celebration in times of joy. May your yoga journey be a source of inspiration, wisdom, and deep connection throughout the many seasons of your life.

Thank you for joining this exploration of yoga essentials. May your practice be a continuous source of strength, peace, and joy, both on and off the mat. As you step forward into the vast landscape of your yoga journey, may it be a journey filled with love, light, and the boundless potential that yoga has to offer.